How To Look More Beautiful And Attractive

347 Foolproof Beauty Tips That Will Make You Look Instantly Better

ADAM COLTON

Published by BizMove
www.bizmove.com

347 Foolproof Beauty Tips That Will Make You Look Instantly Better

When you want to be more beautiful to others, you have to start learning just how you can maximize your beauty routine. Something else to consider is the selection process of both techniques and products that assist you in looking better. Check out the tips in this article to get started.

1. Instead of simply applying lipstick directly to your lips from the tube, invest in a good lip brush. This allows you to create a more well-defined shape that does not smear or smudge around the mouth. Pucker up, then pull your finger through your lips to prevent any lipstick from smudging on your teeth.

2. Never go to the cosmetics counter for skincare application tips while your skin is irritated, bumpy, or in especially bad shape. Applying a new cosmetic product over the irritated skin can actually make the condition much worse. Wait until the condition has improved, then make the trip and set up an appointment.

3. Consuming large quantities of water each day can help you keep your skin looking great without having to buy expensive products. Water will

keep your whole body, including your skin, hydrated. It also can flush harmful toxins from the body, and this action gives you cleaner and healthier skin.

4. Mix your foundation with a moisturizer, as it will stretch the life of your foundation. This will help your skin to glow and add some SPF as well.

5. For beautiful hair, add oil to your hair care routine. You can make your hair shinier, less frizzy, and mask graying by adding a few drops of oil to your hair every morning. Good oils to use are castor, rosemary, or sesame oils. All of them are cost effective and widely available.

6. If your hair is greasy or oily, an easy way to fix this if you don't have time to wash it, is to use a bronzer compact or baby powder. Brunettes should carry bronzer compact and add to extra oily hair, and blondes should do the same with baby powder. This will temporarily hide your unwashed hair.

7. Always apply a heat protectant spray to your hair before using a curling iron, flat iron or hair dryer. Heat can damage your hair, leaving it brittle, dry and full of split ends. Just like their name implies, heat protectant sprays coat your hair to protect it

from the heat. This allows it to stay smooth, sleek and shiny no matter how you choose to style your hair.

8. Add plenty of fruits and vegetables to your diet to make your skin more beautiful. Eating more fruits and vegetables have benefits to every aspect of your health, not just to your skin. Raw food can not just make your skin beautiful and youthful, it can extend your life by years.

9. Here is a beauty tip! Warm your concealer before using it! Often when you put concealer on it can come off looking thick and caked. You have to know how to conceal your concealer. First warm it by rubbing it in circular motion on the back of your hand! Then use your finger to apply.

10. If you have skin that tends to get shiny, you can do one of two things throughout the day. If you want to be fancy, you can buy a packet of face-blotting sheets. These smell wonderful and are impregnated with scented transparent powder. Or you can take a sheet of regular toilet paper and press, not rub, on the oily areas.

11. Your quest for beauty should be a quest to find your best self, not outdo someone else. By being confident in your own innate beauty, you will

exude an air of charm and appeal. You will improve all parts of your life.

12. To help open up smaller eyes, take advantage of the effects of layering your eye makeup. A primer should be applied first and then apply foundation and eye shadow. Once you do this, you should apply a highlighting shadow on your eyes in the inner corners. Use a pencil to apply your eyeliner. You can smudge your eyeliner upward if you wish. This can help make your eyes look their best!

13. Is your face tired looking? Does it need some radiance? With just the swirl of a brush you can instantly brighten up your skin. Illuminating powder is an amazing product that will wake up your skin. Apply it to your face, on the cheekbones, temples, on the chin and under your eye brows. You can wear this alone or over foundation.

14. As part of your beauty routine, buy high quality makeup brushes. High quality brushes contain fine hairs, which will make your cosmetic application even. They are also soft on the skin, so you can avoid those micro scratches that can lead to wrinkles and blemishes. A high quality set

will cost more, but it is well worth the investment.

15. If you love the brightness of red lipstick, but hate how it looks when it smears, then you should keep some makeup remover handy. If the dreaded smear ever happens, use a cotton ball or tissue dipped in makeup remover to erase the stain. Now you won't have to worry what color lipstick you choose for the day.

16. If you want that shiny look on your legs, but don't want a greasy feel to them, just use your regular lotion, and gloss it up a little by adding a small drop of baby oil. This will give you luster and softness, without the resulting greasiness of the baby oil alone.

17. If you have ever had the problem of your eyeliner smearing or crumbling as you try to apply it, try putting it in the freezer for about 15 minutes before you need to use it. This will firm up the tip so the eyeliner goes on smoothly, and you won't have the resulting crumbles or smears.

18. Disposable mascara wands, which are often known by makeup artists as "spoolies", are a cheap and effective tool for your makeup kit. These tiny brushes are useful to break up clumps

in the lashes and brush off excess mascara without spoiling your makeup. In a pinch, they can also be used to groom your eyebrows. They should be disposed after each use.

19. No matter what your skin looks and feels like, it is important to wash your face at least once a day. No matter what you do, take off all your makeup before you clean your skin. If you do not remove all the makeup first, your pores can clog, causing breakouts.

20. Gently brush your lips with a soft toothbrush. This will help you remove dead skin cells from your lips and make them soft. You should then apply Vaseline or another type of lip balm to moisturize your lips and keep them soft. You can do this every day or every other day.

21. Sugaring and waxing cause your hair follicles to open, which can cause many skin problems when exposed to tanning. If you do not wait, you could incur intense irritations. Also, avoid scented products after waxing or sugaring, as it can cause irritation as well.

22. Use a face mask at least once a week. Depending on which one you choose, this will help remove impurities from your face. A mud or clay mask is

best for removing impurities. You will see results immediately. Once you find a mask you like, you should stick with it.

23. If your facial appearance is more square-shaped, use a coral or creamy rose blush which make your face look softer and appear less angular. Apply the creamy blush to the apples of your cheeks with your fingers. Gently tug them and fan the color towards your temples.

24. Consuming large quantities of water each day can help you keep your skin looking great without having to buy expensive products. Water can help flush toxins and wastes out of the body. Not only is it good for your skin, it is good for your health as well.

25. Use a misting spray to set makeup. After you are finished fully making up your face, lightly mist yourself with a sprayer. This will set your makeup, keeping it in place longer before requiring you to touch it up. This is perfect for long nights out or events such as weddings.

26. Make your skin more beautiful by eating fruit. If you have a sweet tooth, and satiate it with sugar, you can quickly see it on your skin. You can feed your sweet tooth, and your skin, by eating sweet

fruit in place of anything sugary. When you do this, your skin won't be the only beneficiary.

27. Remember that fragrance rises. Scents rise. When applying perfume or scented body mist, put it lower on your body. Do not apply too much by putting a little everywhere. Just apply a little around your ankles. The scent will rise without being as overpowering as some perfumes tend to be.

28. If you love a certain nail polish, and it starts to look a little dry or is about to run out, add a little bit of nail polish remover to the bottle. Shake it very well, and you will end up with having an easier time getting some more use out of it.

29. Using a fake tanning lotion can make your skin appear more beautiful without getting any of the harmful rays from sunbathing or tanning. Make sure to shave or wax any hair that you don't want on your body before applying any type of tanning lotion at least 24 hours ahead of time.

30. Paint your toenails before you go to bed. Make sure you have given your nail polish plenty of time to dry before going to bed. When you shower in the morning you can easily peel off

any excess polish that you get on your toes for that perfect manicured look.

31. Kitchen sponges are perfectly fine to use in the bathtub. They work as well as ones specifically designed for the bathroom, and you can buy them in large quantities to save some cash.

32. You can save a lot of money by trimming your own bangs at home. First, make sure you have the proper scissors. Spend the money for a small pair of good haircutting scissors. Trim your bangs dry. How to trim them will depend on your hair type, but most people do best by dividing the bangs into three sections, holding the hair up in a twist, and taking small diagonal snips so that the cuts aren't straight. Drop the twist, see how you look, and repeat until it's short enough for your liking.

33. When you are down to the last drop of your favorite, discontinued shade of nail polish, add a few drops of polish remover to your bottle. Shake it, and then use it in the same way you normally would. The color is going to be a bit clearer, but it is basically the same.

34. Baking soda is your beauty friend. Baking soda is one of those products that you should always

have on hand. For beauty you can use it to make your shampoo work better, whiten your teeth, and cure the pain of sunburn. All of this from one box that hardly costs a dollar.

35. Have you ever had makeup smudges and want an easy way to fix them without re-doing your whole look? Then try a cotton swab and some eye-makeup remover. This way, you can precisely clean up the area you need to re-do when time doesn't allow starting over from scratch.

36. Be sure to exfoliate your face on a regular basis. Exfoliate your skin every other day to keep the top layer looking fresh and smooth. You will ensure you face looks healthier and you will get rid of any dirt or oil build up.

37. If you have fine lines around your eyes, mouth, and forehead, you should look for cosmetics with light-reflecting particles. These products, which are just more matte than shimmery, can reflect light in a way that appears to make the fine lines simply disappear. You can use this trick all over your face, or just in your laugh lines.

38. Heat your eyelash curler with your blow dryer. Hold your curler in front of your hair dryer for a few seconds. Be sure to check the temperature

before using it on your eyelashes because it could burn you. Your eyelashes will curl better with a little heat applied to them.

39. Do you find your nails get easily chipped and scratched once they are painted? Using a top coat can help you avoid this. Just make sure to use a true top coat as this is different than a clear polish. Make sure you purchase top coat rather than clear polish.

40. Apply cream to your eyes every night. The skin around your eyes is delicate, and not as thick as the skin elsewhere on your face. This makes the skin around your eyes more prone to be lined and dry. Keeping the skin moist is a simple solution to that beauty problem.

41. Avoid licking your lips. When you constantly lick your lips, rather than become moist, they actually dry out. Try carrying a lip balm or gloss in your pocket or purse, and put it on anytime you feel like doing some licking. You will soon find your lips in beautiful condition.

42. Invest in a good set of makeup brushes for applying your makeup. They may be spendy but, good applicators are critical to create effective makeup applications. If buying retail is outside

your budget, try searching online vendors. You can often find the same quality brushes for much less.

43. To get smaller pores, cut refined sugars from your diet. Eating large amounts of refined sugar enlarges your pores, and can also lead to breakouts. If you have a sweet tooth, try sating your cravings with natural sugars like the ones found in fruit. Your skin will definitely thank you for it!

44. If you ever find yourself relly under time pressure, here's a great tip on how to do a quick makeup job. Put some waxy lip balm on your fingertip. Then put a dark eyeliner on top of that. Smear it onto your eyes. Then finish with mascara. Apply lipstick. You're ready to go!

45. Using concealer is only half the battle when looking your best and fixing flaws. To have a perfect complexion, try using a lipstick in a warm pink. According to leading makeup artists, no matter what your skin type or tone, warm pink will distract people's eyes from any imperfections and blemishes and keep you looking your best.

46. It is very common to hear the phrase "real beauty comes from within" and this is very true,

even when talking about external beauty. When you feel confident with yourself, it helps you to change many small factors that you may not even realize. The result of this is that you actually look more beautiful, as well.

47. An easy tip for great lips is going glossy. Try putting this on the outside of your lips with some bronzer. Top that with gold or peach-colored gloss.

48. If you're concerned that your freshly painted nails will smear, you can protect them with a thin film of some type of oil. Either put a drop of olive oil on your palm and rub it over the nails, or even easier, use a can of olive oil cooking spray and give each finger just the quickest touch of cooking spray. The oil will form a protective barrier that will keep the polish from smearing.

49. As your skin gets older, be sure to wear the moisturizer that meets your skin's needs for this age. Skin tends to start out oily and becomes drier over time, so it's important to make sure that your skin's need for moisture is being met appropriately. If your moisturizer feels heavy or is giving you skin trouble, it's time to reevaluate.

50. If you are interested in speeding up your metabolism and losing weight as quickly as possible, you should make sure to include ginger in your diet. Ginger, in addition to fighting infections and detoxifying the body, warms you up and increases your body's metabolism rate. Try adding a few slices of ginger to your morning tea and see if it helps you to lose weight.

51. Eyeshadows can be tricky for eyes over 40. Metallic, glittery shadows are beautiful, but eyelid skin develops tiny folds which are, unfortunately, accentuated by those gorgeous metallic colors. On the other hand, some matte shadows look too flat and dry, and do not flatter the eye either. Instead, look for shadows that are neither matte nor metallic: "quietly lustrous" should be the goal.

52. Use steam to refresh your face. Steam releases the impurities in your pores, and you don't need to go to a sauna. A bowl or other container of hot water and a towel are all you need; just hold your head over it and let the piping hot steam redeem your skin.

53. As you get older, exfoliation becomes more and more important to your skin. Use a glycolic acid-rich cream, facial scrub, or even a retinoid gel to

slough off the top layer pf dead skin cells and to reveal the fresh, radiant new skin cells beneath. This can be done three to four times per week for the best effect.

54. Keep your eye gel in your refrigerator. This can help soothe puffy eyes or dark circles around your eyes. Cool eye gel can really make your eyes look refreshed after a long night out. Just apply it as you normally would to see results that are immediate and will last all day.

55. Get an even, natural looking spray tan by investing some time preparing your skin before applying the product. For best results, don't shave or use any other forms of hair removal the day you plan to tan. Exfoliating your skin for several days beforehand will also help you achieve streak free results.

56. Create an alcohol-free natural mouthwash with peppermint oil and purified water. You need one drop of the peppermint oil for each ounce of water. Boil the water, then measure your oil into a glass container that is large enough to hold your mixture. Add the boiling water to the container. Cover the container with a clean cloth (i.e. a handkerchief) and allow to cool. Decant

into a bottle with a tightly fitting lid. Then use this as your mouthwash.

57. A handy beauty tip is to add a little nail polish remover to your nail polish. This helps to thin the nail polish out and make it last a little longer. It is also a good technique to use when your nail polish is a little older and has started to thicken up a bit.

58. When applying eye shadow, look down in the mirror. You should always avoid pulling your eyelids and applying pressure to the lids. Look down when applying your eyeshadow. In this manner, you can see your lids clearly without touching them.

59. To get smaller pores, cut refined sugars from your diet. Eating large amounts of refined sugar enlarges your pores, and can also lead to breakouts. If you have a sweet tooth, try sating your cravings with natural sugars like the ones found in fruit. Your skin will definitely thank you for it!

60. If your favorite color nail polish is getting empty and a bit tacky, add a few drops of nail polish remover to give it new life! You don't have to throw away a half empty bottle of nail lacquer,

just mix in a small amount of regular remover, shake well and your old polish will work like new again.

61. Beauty tip for tired eyes! Eye gel will help reduce the appearance of puffy or tired eyes. Keep this in the refrigerator, and use it for an extra boost if you are really tired. You can feel very tired without having to show it on your face. Just make sure to use the gel on a clean face.

62. If you love the look of powdered mineral makeup but find that it makes your skin itchy, look for a formula that does not contain bismuth oxychloride. This ingredient often irritates skin, but not all brands use it.

63. Immediately after you have applied your lipstick, insert your clean index finger between your lips. Next, remove your finger from your mouth while pursing your lips. This prevents lipstick from moving from the insides of your lips to your teeth without disturbing the lipstick that is on your lips.

64. If you have discovered little white bumps under your eyes, know that these are called Milia and are quite common. They are a harmless form of a cyst caused by dry, dead cells being trapped

under the skin. You can try exfoliation or use a moisturizer that includes an exfoliant with vitamin A to help them disappear, and prevent them in the future.

65. To get rid of white patches on your nails, consume more calcium. The patches are a sign of vitamin deficiency. Clearing up those white spots will allow you to get a smoother and more consistent look with your nail polish. If you can't add more calcium to your diet, start taking a supplement.

66. You can spend big bucks on special dandruff shampoos containing salicylic acid for your dandruff and/or flaky scalp. But did you know that salicylic acid is, in fact, aspirin? So you can skip the expensive shampoos. Just take a regular uncoated aspirin or two, crush it to a powder, and mix it with your shampoo. Let it sit on your scalp for a minute and you will find it has the same result as more expensive treatments.

67. As you grow older, your skin, as a result of sun exposure, becomes darker and is not as light and bright as it was when you were younger. To ensure that your skin remains as bright and lively as possible, make sure that you exfoliate on a

regular basis. Exfoliation will lighten your skin by getting rid of dead skin cells.

68. Open the pores on your face by steaming your face often. It can be done quite easily by filling a bowl with hot water and holding your face over the bowl with a towel over your head. It will open the pores, draw out deep dirt and debris and make your skin glow. Splash your face with cold water directly after to close the pores back up.

69. Consider using baking soda as a means to add some vibrancy to your hair. Mix a little baking soda with your regular amount of shampoo. Then cleanse your tresses normally. This will bring back the luster in your hair.

70. Exfoliate your face and neck at least 2 times a week. Exfoliating helps remove dead skin cells and bring new skin cells to the surface. This will make you look healthy and refreshed when you do this, but you should avoid doing it too much because it can irritate your face.

71. Don't turn the heat up to 11 when taking a bath or shower. In hot water, your pores will open and your skin's natural oils can escape. You are more likely to wash away the oils you need. Wash

yourself with lukewarm water to best take care of your skin. This helps create and maintain soft, supple skin. Also, it will save you on your electricity bill.

72. Eating a spoon of chutney made of curry leaves every day can stop your hair from going gray. This product will help to keep your natural pigment and prevent gray hair from forming. You can also put rosemary essential oil on your locks to achieve a similar effect.

73. For shiny, colorful, rich, beautiful hair, it's important to wash your hair regularly with a good, low-oil shampoo. This is the only way to effectively prevent dandruff and other hair-related ailments. Make sure to also rinse your hair out weekly with apple cider vinegar to wash away chemicals from shampoo.

74. Do not pick or squeeze at your face. A simple beauty rule is to keep your hands off of your face, except to clean or moisturize. You run the risk of causing scars when you pick at your face. You can also transfer oil and dirt onto your face when you are touching it.

75. Do not forget your hands need to be pampered too. Hands are often overlooked in beauty

treatments. That is why it is said, if you want to know someones age, check their hands. In addition to daily treatment with lotion or cream, you should exfoliate your hands once a week.

76. To improve your lip color application, always apply lip balm first. The lip balm will leave your lips soft and moisturized, and will allow your lip color to go on smoothly. Try using a basic, untinted lip balm so that you don't effect the color of the lipstick or lip gloss you're using.

77. For an inexpensive, spa-like facial just lean yourself over a bowl of steaming hot water! Cover or wrap up your hair, fill any container with really hot water and allow the steam to open and clear your pores! It is soothing and stimulating and very cost effective. Follow up with cold water to close and refresh pores, then add moisturizer!

78. If you want to camouflage a pimple, rosacea, a rash or another reddish skin imperfection dab on a green concealer. While it looks strange in the package, the green neutralizes the red tones of irritated skin so you can apply your regular foundation and concealer without the redness showing through.

79. It is essential that you apply a top coat of high-quality to ensure a long- lasting manicure. Put on the topcoat right after you finish the manicure to seal it. Be diligent about applying a touch-up several times a week to ensure that the polish doesn't chip or peel. Your manicure will look fresh and pristine for days longer with the use of a quality top coat.

80. If you have skin that tends to get shiny, you can do one of two things throughout the day. If you want to be fancy, you can buy a packet of face-blotting sheets. These smell wonderful and are impregnated with scented transparent powder. Or you can take a sheet of regular toilet paper and press, not rub, on the oily areas.

81. If you're concerned that your freshly painted nails will smear, you can protect them with a thin film of some type of oil. Either put a drop of olive oil on your palm and rub it over the nails, or even easier, use a can of olive oil cooking spray and give each finger just the quickest touch of cooking spray. The oil will form a protective barrier that will keep the polish from smearing.

82. If you are a woman who is trying to improve your appearance you will want to think about the makeup you use. Remember that like most

things, less is actually more. You don't want to use extreme colors. The idea of makeup is for people to believe that you aren't even using any.

83. If you have an important meeting, take special care with your perfume. Keep the scent light and airy so as not to overwhelm. You should put a small amount behind your ears and on your wrists. This will assure that you smell great when you are hugging and shaking hands at the meeting.

84. Keep some fabric softener sheets on hand for beauty emergencies. Fabric sheets can be used to tame a static skirt that wants to stick you your hose. It can do the same for wild hair. Another thing it is good for is running through your hair to quell obnoxious odors like smoke.

85. Did you get a look at yourself in a public mirror and notice how oily your skin looks? Don't fret. Tear off a corner of toilet paper, and dab it on your skin to soak up the oil and shine. The hard toilet paper is an excellent blotter, and you look picture perfect again.

86. Wear sunscreen to keep your skin protected. Use products with healthy antioxidants. These

items provide nourishment and protect skin, while helping it stay young and supple.

87. Keep your eye gel in your refrigerator. This can help soothe puffy eyes or dark circles around your eyes. Cool eye gel can really make your eyes look refreshed after a long night out. Just apply it as you normally would to see results that are immediate and will last all day.

88. When you nail polish starts to thicken up, you can add a few drops of nail polish remover to the bottle to thin it. Shake the bottle well after the addition of the nail polish remover to mix thoroughly and continue your manicure as usual. You should be able to get several more applications from the bottle.

89. Use a highlighter or moisturizer with warm gold or pink undertones to add some life back to dull wintery skin. Apply this product with a cosmetic sponge to your cheeks and brow bones and experience a radiant effect. Do not do any more than this because you will end up looking shiny.

90. Prolong your foundation by adding a moisturizer into the bottle. The moisturizer makes the foundation lighter so your makeup will not look caked on.

91. Sharpen your eyeliner and lip liner on a regular basis. This keeps them clean and ready to use. If you tend to break your eyeliners when you sharpen them, try placing them in the fridge for a few minutes.

92. You do not need to spend a lot of money on a fancy deep conditioning mask. There are many recipes you can make at home that include foods filled with nutrients that are great for your hair. A great one includes mashed strawberries and enough mayonnaise to make a spreadable paste. Leave it in your wet hair for 10 minutes and rinse.

93. A simple trick to concealing your blemishes is a touch of a red or pink lipstick. No, do not put the lipstick on the flaw itself, but a warm pink lipstick goes with every skin tone and draws the eye to your lips. With a combination of concealer and great looking lips, your blemishes will be hardly noticeable.

94. Give your face a monthly beauty treatment. You do not need to go to a spa to get your skin in its best shape. You can, instead, give yourself a complete facial at home. Start with a product to

exfoliate, follow with a mudpack, next apply an astringent, and finish with a deep moisturizer.

95. To make red lipstick last longer, apply powder and lip liner to your lips before applying the lipstick. First, powder your lips with your usual face powder. Next, draw a line around your lips and fill them in with a red lip liner. Finally, apply the red lipstick on top of the powder and liner, blotting with a tissue to remove any excess lipstick.

96. Exfoliating your body prior to applying tanning lotion or spending time in a tanning bed will extend the life of your tan! Since skin sheds, it's best to do as much of it as possible before getting that great tan so you can keep the glorious glow even longer! Any natural exfoliant applied a day or two before tanning will do!

97. Beauty tip for tired eyes! Eye gel will help reduce the appearance of puffy or tired eyes. Keep this in the refrigerator, and use it for an extra boost if you are really tired. You can feel very tired without having to show it on your face. Just make sure to use the gel on a clean face.

98. People who don't take the following advice are guaranteed to look terrible. Always shape or

pluck your eyebrows to avoid uni-brow. If your eyebrows grow together or even if they are just overly bushy, by trimming them, you will increase your beauty.

99. If you feel as though you are having one off day you shouldn't fret. There are some aspects that are out of your control which will affect your daily appearance. One of the biggest variables is the weather and a humid day can wreck havoc on someone, especially a woman who has larger hair.

100.   When you are trying to improve the quality of your skin, one point that you can never overlook in your routine is a good exfoliation. You should do this at least twice a week and you should have a separate product for your face and your body. These will help to make your skin look younger.

101.   Try tinting your eyebrows when dying your hair. You can do this with a brow pencil on your own, or you can just head over to a salon to get it done. It can help define your face better and make you appear more refreshed and youthful.

102.   Many women get stuck in a look because that's what they get comfortable with. There's

nothing wrong with that, if that's what you like. But, if you have any reason to want a new look, you might want to visit a nice salon and talk to a beauty professional.

103.   Help reduce the appearance of the dark shadows and bags around your eyes by giving yourself a bit of a massage. Use some good moisturizer on your fingertips and massage around the eye area. It assists with lymphatic drainage around your eyes and will reduce the appearance of the damage.

104.   When you file your nails, make sure you don't file in only one direction. This can put stress on your nails and cause them to weaken, become thin and break easily.

105.   Wear gloves when you are applying tanning lotions and keep a towel near you. This will help you if you make a mess and to keep your palms from turning orange or tan. You should also make sure to pull your hair back so your tan is evenly applied.

106.   Instead of simply applying lipstick directly to your lips from the tube, invest in a good lip brush. This allows you to create a more well-defined shape that does not smear or smudge

around the mouth. Pucker up, then pull your finger through your lips to prevent any lipstick from smudging on your teeth.

107.   Make your nail polish last longer. You can make your nails look like you just had a manicure and last longer by using a base coat, 2 coats of color and a top coat. This will provide your nails with a glossy look that will last for at least a few weeks.

108.   Make your skin look more vibrant by using a moisturizer with a warm gold or pink undertone. Apply the highlighter with a makeup sponge, dabbing it on your brows and fleshy part of your cheeks for a dewy look. To keep from looking shiny you should only apply the moisturizer to the apple of your cheeks and underneath your eyebrows.

109.   Consider a new hairstyle for a more narrow-appearing face. Seek cuts featuring long lines and that fall somewhere between the jawline and the shoulders. Bangs and highlights can also do wonders. These ultra-flattering highlights bring attention to your best features.

110.   You can apply makeup to your wide-set eyes in a way that is very flattering and can make the

eyes appear closer together. First, apply a dark brown or navy eyeliner to the inner corners of your eyes, then blend it with a sponge. Apply your eyeshadow at the inner corners, then blend well outward.

111.   If possible, think about buying more than one container of each product you like to use, whether a powder, blush or lip gloss. You should keep them somewhere you can get to them easy. This ensures you always look your best.

112.   Do not forget your hands need to be pampered too. Hands are often overlooked in beauty treatments. That is why it is said, if you want to know someones age, check their hands. In addition to daily treatment with lotion or cream, you should exfoliate your hands once a week.

113.   To make red lipstick last longer, apply powder and lip liner to your lips before applying the lipstick. First, powder your lips with your usual face powder. Next, draw a line around your lips and fill them in with a red lip liner. Finally, apply the red lipstick on top of the powder and liner, blotting with a tissue to remove any excess lipstick.

114.   Curry leaf chutney is a great thing to eat to prevent your hair from going gray. The chutney improves the formation of the pigments that create the color in your hair. One teaspoon a day is enough.

115.   To get even more mileage out of your favorite eye gel, keep it in the refrigerator! The ingredients in eye gel work hard to restore and protect the delicate skin around your eyes and keeping it cold enhances the refreshment factor ten fold! The cold will also work immediately to reduce that dreadful puffiness!

116.   When you are trying to improve the quality of your skin, one point that you can never overlook in your routine is a good exfoliation. You should do this at least twice a week and you should have a separate product for your face and your body. These will help to make your skin look younger.

117.   Very delicate hair, which is prone to frizz, can be damaged by towel drying. A better way to towel-dry is to scrunch your wet hair gently with the towel, then pat it dry to finish. Although it may not provide instant gratification, it will produce noticeably improved results.

118.   If you hate the problems of clumpy and matted eyelashes, try using an eyelash curler. This will make the eyelashes thick and full without using any products. When using the curler, start at the roots and only use on lashes that are clean. Over time your lashes will become fuller, thicker, and beautiful.

119.   Many people tend to get dead skin on their lips. This makes them look old and dry. A great way to prevent this from happening is to brush your lips gently with a toothbrush every single day. After you have done this, you will want to put some balm on to keep them protected.

120.   Crush up an aspirin and put it in your shampoo to get rid of dandruff. This will save you money on buying pricey shampoos made for dandruff. The painkilling properties in aspirin will calm your dry scalp and get rid of dandruff problems while using your favorite shampoo and conditioner.

121.   Give yourself a mini facial using a mask made from an egg white and a dash of lemon juice. Leave the mask on for about two minutes, and then rinse. This gives your skin an instant tightening effect and is ideal to do about an hour before an evening out on the town.

122. As you get older, exfoliation becomes more and more important to your skin. Use a glycolic acid-rich cream, facial scrub, or even a retinoid gel to slough off the top layer pf dead skin cells and to reveal the fresh, radiant new skin cells beneath. This can be done three to four times per week for the best effect.

123. A coat or two of waterproof black or dark brown mascara is an easy way to open up the eyes and draw attention to them. Concentrate on the edges of your eyes by using mascara wands to open up masses of makeup that have clumped together.

124. An odd but great trick is to apply Vaseline to your eyebrows right before you head to bed. This will help your brows to be nice and shiny. Be sure to focus the Vaseline only on your brows, as getting this on your skin can cause acne.

125. To give your medium-to long-length hair a quick boost of volume in the morning, turn your head upside down, then apply a spray-on product like mousse or serum to add volume. Aim for the roots, then scrunch your hair at the crown and sides. Turn right-side up, then use your fingers to smooth the top layer.

126.   Wear gloves when you are applying tanning lotions and keep a towel near you. This will help you if you make a mess and to keep your palms from turning orange or tan. You should also make sure to pull your hair back so your tan is evenly applied.

127.   Have some Vitamin E around. This vitamin can be used in different ways. Vitamin E will help keep your skin looking smooth and soft. Vitamin E is also an effective way to soften cuticles.

128.   Create the illusion of less deep-set eyes by using lightly colored eyeshadow to the entire eyelid. The light colors will appear to come forward, whereas a darker liner or shadow would have the reverse affect, making the eyes appear to recede further into the face. The color you apply should be light and very subtle.

129.   To determine whether you have cool or warm skin tones, check out the veins on the inside of your wrist. If you have cool skin, the veins will appear bluish in color. If you have warm skin, they will have a greenish tint instead. Cool skin tones look best in cool colors, such as

blue and purple, whereas warm skin tones, look best in warm colors like red, yellow and orange.

130.   Your skin is constantly changing from day to day based upon your age, hormone levels, climate, and even our daily activities. As a result, you should be aware that your skincare and beauty regimen should be flexible enough to change in order to adapt to the needs of your skin.

131.   Add plenty of fruits and vegetables to your diet to make your skin more beautiful. Eating more fruits and vegetables have benefits to every aspect of your health, not just to your skin. Raw food can not just make your skin beautiful and youthful, it can extend your life by years.

132.   Many people find honey to be great for natural beauty treatments. Honey can really benefit your skin when consumed. When exfoliating your skin, mix honey with sugar. If you put honey in your moisturizer, it will help you retain it. If you add honey to your shampoo, it will make your hair soft and shiny.

133.   Pick a matte blush instead of a shimmer blush, unless you do not have any flaws on your skin. Shimmer blushes can bring out blemishes

and imperfections like scars and acne. However, matte blushes help to hide blemishes, so that your skin looks flawless and radiant.

134.   Pat moisturizer into your skin instead of rubbing it. Most people rub their moisturizer into their skin. This can actually disperse the moisturizer to different parts of your skin or even remove most of it entirely. Try patting it over your skin instead. Your skin will absorb it more evenly.

135.   If you ever find yourself relly under time pressure, here's a great tip on how to do a quick makeup job. Put some waxy lip balm on your fingertip. Then put a dark eyeliner on top of that. Smear it onto your eyes. Then finish with mascara. Apply lipstick. You're ready to go!

136.   Smoking, besides being linked to a myriad of health problems, also has an extremely negative affect on the way you look. One of the best beauty tips is to never smoke a cigarette in your life, and if you are a smoker, stop immediately. Smoking prematurely ages the skin and causes wrinkles, it makes acne worse and it turns your teeth yellow.

137.   Mineral powder makeup is very popular and looks great but can cause irritation because many formulations contain bismuth oxychloride. This irritates skin, so women think they can't use this kind of makeup. However, a lot of brands don't use that ingredient.

138.   Use a cleansing shampoo at least once a week. Your hair gets all sorts of buildup on it and the normal shampoo does help, but nothing really cleanses it better then a cleansing shampoo. After you do this, you will notice that your hair just feels softer and lighter. It also looks better too.

139.   Enhance your eyes by doing work on your eyelashes. Many women just apply mascara and go on their way. If you take the additional second to curl your eyelashes prior to applying the mascara, you will accentuate the eyes better than you would if you just apply the mascara.

140.   If you are light skinned or have light hair you may want to consider tinting your eyebrows. This will enhance the color of your eyebrows and will draw attention to your eyes and brows. You can tint your eyebrows by yourself and can find the the tint at most beauty stores.

141.   Eyeliner can add impact in a way that few products can. Steady your elbow on the table to avoid making mistakes, then use an eye pencil with a dull point to draw on a series of small dashes across the upper lash line. Use a smudging tool or sponge to blend the dashes to create a single line.

142.   Prior to putting on your makeup, apply some light moisturizer. While moisturizers are excellent for your skin, they also aid in spreading your makeup evenly. If you apply makeup without a moisturizer, you might appear blotchy. This trick is also great at extending the wearing time of your makeup and keeping you looking fresh.

143.   A fluffy brush and a dusting of matte powder are all it takes to freshen up your makeup if you need to go from daytime to night. You can enhance your cheeks by using some shimmery powder on them.

144.   Darkening very light eyelashes can really open up the eyes and make a noticeable impact on the eye color. Avoid using black mascara, which may appear way too harsh on light lashes and against lighter hair colors. Instead, you can

have them tinted professionally or you can use brown pencil to line your eyes.

145.   Avoid licking your lips. When you constantly lick your lips, rather than become moist, they actually dry out. Try carrying a lip balm or gloss in your pocket or purse, and put it on anytime you feel like doing some licking. You will soon find your lips in beautiful condition.

146.   It is always a good idea to select a matte blush instead of a shimmer blush unless your skin is flawless. Shimmer blushes can bring out blemishes and imperfections like scars and acne. Matte blushes, on the other hand, can camouflage blemishes, helping to give you the look of radiant, flawless skin.

147.   Keep to a schedule for maximum beauty benefit. You do not have to schedule everything, but you do need to schedule your meals. Studies have shown that people who are consistent with their routines concerning food and drink, look years younger, and live longer, than people who are sporadic with their eating times.

148.   Create a funky, modern nail design by using scrapbooking scissors with scalloped, zig-zag or other edges. You can cut regular cellophane tape

with the scissors and place them on your nails before painting to create great stripes, two-tone effects, or other interesting designs. Try using matte polishes next to glossy ones for a multi-textured effect.

149.   Whiten your teeth using strawberries. Before a big event or pictures and to instantly whiten your teeth, use the juicy side of a cut strawberry and rub over your teeth. This will help whiten them quickly and easily. This works great if you are unprepared or running low on time.

150.   Many women like to use concealer under their foundation. If you've run out of concealer, or can't find it, look inside the cap of your foundation. Liquid and lotion foundations tend to collect and thicken inside the cap and will work well in a pinch as an emergency concealer.

151.   Once you have found a haircolor you like, be sure to buy an extra box or two of it to keep at home. That way, you will never be out of the color you like if they happen to run out of it at the local drugstore or beauty center.

152.   When painting your nails, always use a good base coat. Not only does a base coat allow polish to better adhere to your nails, but it prevents

your nails from becoming discolored, which is common when using darker colors. For maximum staying power, look for adhesive base coats, which dry to a somewhat tacky finish.

153.   When it comes to enhancing your natural beauty, it helps to start from within. The proper knowledge is often the only difference between people who have an attractive and well-groomed appearance and people who lack this refined presentation. Once you become informed on the appropriate self-care methods, improving your appearance will seem much less complicated.

154.   Facial skin-tightening help is as close as ingredients found in your refrigerator! Put together some egg whites and lemon and then rinse it off in a few minutes. This is perfect to do before you have a blind date, for example.

155.   During hairstyling, start from the back forwards and work section to section. The back is the hardest area to work (and will take the most time) because it is the hardest to reach. When you blow your hair dry, your arms can get tired, so start with the hardest part first.

156.   The mouth is the ultimate attention getter. If you wear lipstick, know that the color you wear

can work for or against you. Choose a color that compliments your skin and that is "in" for the season and you will look amazing. If you want to help your lipstick last longer, apply powder over the first coat and then reapply. If you don't wear lipstick, make sure your lips are well hydrated and you regularly use chapstick. Chapped cracked lips will detract from your appearance.

157.   Used coffee grounds are a great way to exfoliate for your hands. Once cooled, put the coffee grounds in a plastic bag, and keep them in the refrigerator. Rub about a teaspoon of grounds a couple of times a week, then rinse, and apply hand cream as usual. Coffee grounds work in much the same way as when you exfoliate with sand-based products, and your hands will feel silky smooth.

158.   You can protect yourself immensely from the sun by using sunscreen. Use products with healthy antioxidants. These skin care ingredients give nourishment and protection to your skin, helping it maintain its suppleness and youthful look.

159.   Apply a moisturizer that is light before putting a fake tan on your skin. A fake tan will collect on spots of your skin that are dry. You

should make sure you pay attention to your feet, elbows, knees and around your wrists. Apply lotion to these areas before applying a fake tanner.

160.   Take your time applying a fake tan. Make sure you have at least 30 minutes before going to bed or getting dressed. If you are in a hurry then wait to do it because you may get streaky results. It is important to make sure you properly apply a fake tan.

161.   Find the perfect makeup for yourself. With so many different types to choose from look for makeup that is noncomedogenic. Avoid trying too many different types of makeup because this can irritate your skin. Instead, find one that works for you and stick with it.

162.   Use lukewarm water to cleanse your face when bathing. The hot water will open your pores, exposing the natural skin oils that hold in moisture. You are more likely to wash away the oils you need. Go for lukewarm water, not hot water, for the best results in keeping your skin luxuriously soft. Also, it will save you on your electricity bill.

163.　Drink milk on a daily basis. Everyone knows that drinking will make your skin and bones much healthier. Milk has a lot of protein and builds muscles. It can also help you shed some weight. Consume at least one glass of milk if you want to keep your health and beauty.

164.　In order to make your teeth look whiter, use lipstick with cool, blue undertones. Lipsticks with warm, orange-based undertones accentuate the natural yellow color of your teeth, making them look yellower. Lipsticks with cool, blue-based undertones, on the other hand, will make your teeth look whiter. For the greatest impact, choose a bright red lipstick with blue undertones.

165.　Always remove makeup before going to bed. If you sleep with your makeup on, you increase the likelihood you will get acne and blackheads. Makeup can trap dirt and oil on your face. Clean and tone your face every night. Don't forget to add moisturizer when you are finished cleaning.

166.　Petroleum jelly is the best way to keep the skin on your feet soft and supple. There are thousands of lotions and creams for your feet but they can be expensive and may have negative effects. Use it up to three times a week on your feet to prevent chaffing, peeling, and to leave your feel smooth and soft.

167.   Beauty tip for tired eyes! Eye gel will help reduce the appearance of puffy or tired eyes. Keep this in the refrigerator, and use it for an extra boost if you are really tired. You can feel very tired without having to show it on your face. Just make sure to use the gel on a clean face.

168.   Sometimes, when coloring your hair, you may find that the color you chose simply isn't strong or intense enough for your liking. You can solve this problem by purchasing a second box of color, mixing half the product with shampoo, and reapplying it to just-colored hair. Let it sit for only 5-10 minutes before rinsing and you will find the color intensified.

169.   A proven solution to dead skin buildup is to use a pumice stone in the shower. The skin is much softer when it absorbs moisture from the shower so it will come off easier. Do not use a razor to remove dead skin, this causes more skin to grow back in the areas which it was removed.

170.   Beauty is in the details, so you may have to spend a little bit of time on the small things that

are often overlooked. This could mean using a good exfoliant in the shower or learning the correct way to shave your face or your legs. These small things add up to a much better you.

171.   If you want a dramatic look for your eyes, try a liquid eyeliner. You have more space for creativity with liquid and it will enhance your eyes. When it comes to picking a brush out, be sure it is small and its bristles are angled for ideal results.

172.   If you find that your feet are dry and scaly looking and feeling, try using a petroleum jelly product to treat them. Apply a generous amount on your feet and cover them with thick socks at night before you go to bed. Your feet will absorb the moisture out of the petroleum jelly and will quickly look and feel much better.

173.   You can spend big bucks on special dandruff shampoos containing salicylic acid for your dandruff and/or flaky scalp. But did you know that salicylic acid is, in fact, aspirin? So you can skip the expensive shampoos. Just take a regular uncoated aspirin or two, crush it to a powder, and mix it with your shampoo. Let it sit on your scalp for a minute and you will find it has the same result as more expensive treatments.

174. Eyeliner can add impact in a way that few products can. Steady your elbow on the table to avoid making mistakes, then use an eye pencil with a dull point to draw on a series of small dashes across the upper lash line. Use a smudging tool or sponge to blend the dashes to create a single line.

175. If you have problems keeping wild and unruly brows tamed, you can keep them under control by spraying a brow brush with a bit of hairspray or clear brow gel, then gently combing your brows into place. For added shaping, you can even use a very small dab of Vaseline.

176. Apply eye shadow to seal in eyeliner. When you are making up your eyes, apply your liner before your eye shadow. Then, when applying the shadow, slightly dampen a cotton swab and add some eye shadow. Smooth this over the liner and you will find it lasts much longer.

177. Always apply a heat protectant spray to your hair before using a curling iron, flat iron or hair dryer. Heat can damage your hair, leaving it brittle, dry and full of split ends. Just like their name implies, heat protectant sprays coat your hair to protect it from the heat. This allows it to

stay smooth, sleek and shiny no matter how you choose to style your hair.

178.   A great tip to use when tweezing your eyebrows is to use restrain. Over plucking the brows can lead to bald patches and emaciated brows where hair only grows back irregularly. If this has happened, use a brow gel which is protein-spiked to encourage healthy regrowth and brow fillers that can shade in areas that are problems.

179.   When painting your nails, always use a good base coat. Not only does a base coat allow polish to better adhere to your nails, but it prevents your nails from becoming discolored, which is common when using darker colors. For maximum staying power, look for adhesive base coats, which dry to a somewhat tacky finish.

180.   Beauty is in the details, so you may have to spend a little bit of time on the small things that are often overlooked. This could mean using a good exfoliant in the shower or learning the correct way to shave your face or your legs. These small things add up to a much better you.

181.   Make sure you both shave and then exfoliate prior to any application of a tanning spray.

Proper skin preparation ensures an even coating of color, making the end result look more natural.

182. For soft feet, apply lotion or Vaseline and wrap in cling wrap before going to bed. You should then put socks on your feet. You should do this at least once a week for the softest feet. This will prepare even the driest feet for summer and wearing sandals.

183. Keep petroleum jelly on hand for a variety of beauty tricks. Use it for removing eye make-up, it is gentle and effective. Use it as an intensive dry skin treatment. Use petroleum jelly in place of lip gloss for healthy soft lips. It is widely available and cost effective.

184. Many people tend to get dead skin on their lips. This makes them look old and dry. A great way to prevent this from happening is to brush your lips gently with a toothbrush every single day. After you have done this, you will want to put some balm on to keep them protected.

185. The mouth is the ultimate attention getter. If you wear lipstick, know that the color you wear can work for or against you. Choose a color that compliments your skin and that is "in" for the

season and you will look amazing. If you want to
help your lipstick last longer, apply powder over
the first coat and then reapply. If you don't wear
lipstick, make sure your lips are well hydrated
and you regularly use chapstick. Chapped
cracked lips will detract from your appearance.

186.   Use the ignition part of a matchbook or box
if you don't have a nail file. If you find yourself
in need of a nail file, but can't seem to find one,
you can use the rough part you use to light
matches on a match book as a nail file.

187.   If your eyebrows have become a bit unruly
and you want to tame them, try using a small
amount of hair spray on them. What you would
do is get an eyebrow comb or unused
toothbrush, and spray it with the hair spray.
Comb through the brows to flatten and smooth
them.

188.   Finding a new hair style that is different
from what one usually does with their hair can
not only give one a fresh look but enhance their
beauty. A new hair style can attract attention
from people who notice the difference and also
frame ones face in a new way that may enhance
beauty.

189.   If you are trying to reduce the puffiness around your eyes try holding a cold spoon on the puffy areas. The cold can cause the puffiness to go away making your face look more beautiful.

190.   Take care of your teeth. A beautiful smile can brighten your appearance just as much as a terrible smile can hurt your appearance. Make sure to have dental checkups as well as to fix any cosmetic dental problems that make you feel uncomfortable. Being happy with your smile will show on your face; it will make you look that much better.

191.   If you need to soak up extra oil in your T-Zones, you can use blotting papers to quickly give your face a more matte appearance. These sheets often come in small, pocket-sized packets; many are offered with rice powder or in a powder-free option. The packets are very cheap and can be slipped into your purse or desk drawer.

192.   According to scientific studies, quite a few people find beauty in symmetry. Taking steps to improve the symmetry of your face can make you appear more attractive. Make your makeup, beard and mustache identical and symmetrical on both the right and left sides.

193.   Use eye drops to liven up your face. Tired eyes can bring down your whole look. Keep a small bottle of eye drops in your bag and use them periodically, especially when sitting in front of your computer. They will not only freshen up your eyes, but make them sparkle too.

194.   Do you find that your nails become chipped and scratched after each manicure? Try a top coat, which will help your nails stay shiny and glossy for up to 7 days! Be certain you do not confuse this product with typical clear polishes, as they do differ quite a bit. Buy top coat, not clear polish.

195.   A handy beauty tip is to add a little nail polish remover to your nail polish. This helps to thin the nail polish out and make it last a little longer. It is also a good technique to use when your nail polish is a little older and has started to thicken up a bit.

196.   To make red lipstick last longer, apply powder and lip liner to your lips before applying the lipstick. First, powder your lips with your usual face powder. Next, draw a line around your lips and fill them in with a red lip liner. Finally, apply the red lipstick on top of the powder and

liner, blotting with a tissue to remove any excess lipstick.

197.   To extend the life of your lip gloss, apply a lip liner first. Be sure to match your lip shade with the lip liner. By taking this step first you're gloss will be sure to stay on much longer.

198.   Choose your eyeshadow based on your eye color to make your eye makeup really pop. If your eyes are blue, shades of brown are the most flattering. For brown eyes, try purple shadows like lavender or plum. If your eyes are green, golden shades are very flattering, as are many shades from the brown family.

199.   If you suffer from hair loss or brittle hair it may be caused by a poor diet and a lack of essential nutrients. In order to ensure that your hair is strong and healthy consider supplementing your diet with the following vitamins: Iron, Vitamin A, Vitamin H, Vitamin B5, Vitamin E and Zinc.

200.   Give the glossy look a try; it is the one of the simplest ways to keep your lips beautiful and lusciously full. First, outline the lip edges a few shades darker than your actual skin tone using a

concealer brush and bronzer. Top that with a glossy shade of coral, gold or peach.

201.   If you have discovered little white bumps under your eyes, know that these are called Milia and are quite common. They are a harmless form of a cyst caused by dry, dead cells being trapped under the skin. You can try exfoliation or use a moisturizer that includes an exfoliant with vitamin A to help them disappear, and prevent them in the future.

202.   When looking at beauty products, you should always be sure to check out as many reviews as possible. Sometimes it is not worth it to spend a lot for a product when you can purchase the same type of product for much less. Other times it is essential that you spend the extra money to get the right product.

203.   You can spend big bucks on special dandruff shampoos containing salicylic acid for your dandruff and/or flaky scalp. But did you know that salicylic acid is, in fact, aspirin? So you can skip the expensive shampoos. Just take a regular uncoated aspirin or two, crush it to a powder, and mix it with your shampoo. Let it sit on your scalp for a minute and you will find it has the same result as more expensive treatments.

204.   When applying make up you want to be sure that you do it in a gentle way. If you use strokes that are too strong you can have two problems. The first of these is that the abrasive nature of the strokes can damage your skin. Secondly, it leads to a lack of control and worse makeup.

205.   If you are over a certain age and uncertain as to how to wear makeup in a flattering way, please take advantage of the makeup professionals at your local department store. Pick a brand that appeals to you and plunk yourself down in the chair of the most skilled-looking makeup artist. They will be happy to give you tons of free helpful advice on the best way to bring your "now" beauty out. Whether you buy their products or not is entirely up to you, but the makeover and the advice are free and yours to keep.

206.   If you are interested in speeding up your metabolism and losing weight as quickly as possible, you should make sure to include ginger in your diet. Ginger, in addition to fighting infections and detoxifying the body, warms you up and increases your body's metabolism rate. Try adding a few slices of ginger to your morning tea and see if it helps you to lose weight.

207.   You can put your moisturizer in an empty jar or tube of lip gloss. You could stash the portable container in a purse, travel bag or in a desk drawer at your work. You can use a quick dab of it to counteract feelings of dryness as soon as they occur.

208.   Try rubbing Vaseline onto your feet before bed. Your feet will feel as smooth as a baby's bottom. You can add this to your nightly beauty ritual to make it easier to remember. Apply your Vaseline liberally and then slip on your socks as they will keep it on your feet and off your sheets!

209.   If you want to add a pinch of color to your face midday, consider stocking up on a stick of cream blush or a gel-based cheek blusher. Apply a small amount to the apples of your cheek, then blending in circular motions. This keeps your face looking fresh in a natural and easily applied in a manner that is especially flattering.

210.   Look for a concealer palette that comes with two different shades of concealer. This allows you to blend a perfectly customized shade that will melt flawlessly into your skin. Use small dabbing and patting motions to apply the

concealer over red areas, broken capillaries, and any other marks or discolored areas.

211.   A few drops of rich sweet almond oil can be a very useful addition to your skincare routine as well as for use in emergencies. Use it on dry skin to infuse heavy duty moisture, or apply it to your cuticles to make them noticeably softer before a manicure or pedicure.

212.   Red eyes make you look tired and worn out. Carry a bottle of eye drops in your purse and reapply as needed throughout the day. At home, keep a bottle of eye drops in the refrigerator to refresh your eyes when you get home from a day in a dry, air conditioned office.

213.   Cracked heels and dry, flaking feet are very unattractive, especially in sandals. To combat this problem, right before you go to bed, soak your feet in a warm water bath for ten minutes, coat them with petroleum jelly and then cover them with a thick pair of socks to lock in the moisture. In no time, you'll have soft feet.

214.   If you are looking for some individualized attention from a cosmetics salesperson, visit the mall or department store during the early morning or daytime during the week. If you go

on the weekend, your consultant will not be able to give you a thorough assessment and unhurried cosmetics application.

215.   Pick a foundation that is dermatologist approved and matches your natural skin tone well. Some foundations can clog your pores quite easily if you have sensitive skin, so find one that is oil-free as well. This will help keep your pores clear and help make your face look great and oil-free all day.

216.   Keep your skin, body, hair and nails looking great by eating a healthy, well-balanced diet. Providing your body with the vitamins and nutrients it needs is the most effective way to look your best. So, remember that beauty starts with healthy food choices while shopping for groceries.

217.   Most women would be surprised to know that the average female devotes more than 60 hours of her life to the ordeal of shaving and waxing. Laser hair removal, while somewhat costly, will save you a great deal of time and nicks on your legs, underarm, face, and bikini area.

218.   Do not pick or squeeze at your face. A simple beauty rule is to keep your hands off of your face, except to clean or moisturize. You run the risk of causing scars when you pick at your face. You can also transfer oil and dirt onto your face when you are touching it.

219.   Avoid refined foods as part of your daily beauty routine. Refined foods take away most of the nutrients that would naturally be found in a food. Often times the good things are replaced by chemicals and fortifiers. Your overall health will vastly improve, not just your skin, nails, and hair.

220.   To make red lipstick last longer, apply powder and lip liner to your lips before applying the lipstick. First, powder your lips with your usual face powder. Next, draw a line around your lips and fill them in with a red lip liner. Finally, apply the red lipstick on top of the powder and liner, blotting with a tissue to remove any excess lipstick.

221.   Go on a detox diet once a month to maximize your beauty routine. You may not realize how many toxins are building up in your body on a daily basis. If you do not remove them

regularly, they just sit in your body, and may later negatively affect your health.

222.   Once you have found a haircolor you like, be sure to buy an extra box or two of it to keep at home. That way, you will never be out of the color you like if they happen to run out of it at the local drugstore or beauty center.

223.   When looking at beauty products, you should always be sure to check out as many reviews as possible. Sometimes it is not worth it to spend a lot for a product when you can purchase the same type of product for much less. Other times it is essential that you spend the extra money to get the right product.

224.   Choose a dark mascara to attract attention to your eyes and make them seem larger. Use disposable mascara wands for eliminating clumps and extra mascara from the outer edges of the eyes.

225.   Instead of simply applying lipstick directly to your lips from the tube, invest in a good lip brush. This allows you to create a more well-defined shape that does not smear or smudge around the mouth. Pucker up, then pull your

finger through your lips to prevent any lipstick from smudging on your teeth.

226.   Since unwanted facial hair can be embarrassing, remove it. You can easily do this yourself by using wax or tweezers. Or, you can have it done at a salon by a professional. Either way is an easy solution to help you feel better about your appearance.

227.   To keep feet looking beautiful, especially during the warmer, dryer summer months, try applying Vaseline to them every day. It will keep them smooth and soft. Then go get yourself a pedicure and a pair of brand new sassy sandals, and you'll have the best looking feet of the season.

228.   To determine whether you have cool or warm skin tones, check out the veins on the inside of your wrist. If you have cool skin, the veins will appear bluish in color. If you have warm skin, they will have a greenish tint instead. Cool skin tones look best in cool colors, such as blue and purple, whereas warm skin tones, look best in warm colors like red, yellow and orange.

229.   For a torn or split fingernail, use a teabag if you can't run to the salon to fix it. You need to

take the tea from the teabag first. Then, cut a piece of the teabag that is the size of the tear. Simply, place your patch over the tear and coat the entire nail, including the patch, with nail strengthener or clear nail polish.

230.   To make your eyelashes look thicker, dust them with a coat of loose powder before applying your mascara. Use a small brush to apply a thin layer of translucent powder to your eyelashes, taking care not to get the powder in your eyes. Follow up with a coat of your favorite mascara over the top of the powder.

231.   Here is a beauty tip! Warm your concealer before using it! Often when you put concealer on it can come off looking thick and caked. You have to know how to conceal your concealer. First warm it by rubbing it in circular motion on the back of your hand! Then use your finger to apply.

232.   To highlight your eyes and make them look larger and more awake, use a shimmery, pale shade of vanilla or light gold just under your brow bone. You can sweep it down to cover your entire lid for a natural look, or sweep it on after applying your other eye colors to frame your eyes.

233.   To give more definition to your eyes apply mascara. If you only have a few minutes, you can apply mascara to highlight your eyes, and look like you have spent more time than you really have getting ready. Adding eye color will only take a few moments, and really completes your look.

234.   To get rid of white patches on your nails, consume more calcium. The patches are a sign of vitamin deficiency. Clearing up those white spots will allow you to get a smoother and more consistent look with your nail polish. If you can't add more calcium to your diet, start taking a supplement.

235.   Enhance your eyes by doing work on your eyelashes. Many women just apply mascara and go on their way. If you take the additional second to curl your eyelashes prior to applying the mascara, you will accentuate the eyes better than you would if you just apply the mascara.

236.   If you want to fill in your brows but find pencils too harsh-looking, try a brow powder that's a bit lighter than your hair color. Powder provides a softer look and is easier to blend than

waxy pencils. You can set the powder using a brow gel or a dab of clear mascara.

237.   As you grow older, your skin, as a result of sun exposure, becomes darker and is not as light and bright as it was when you were younger. To ensure that your skin remains as bright and lively as possible, make sure that you exfoliate on a regular basis. Exfoliation will lighten your skin by getting rid of dead skin cells.

238.   As part of your beauty routine, buy high quality makeup brushes. High quality brushes contain fine hairs, which will make your cosmetic application even. They are also soft on the skin, so you can avoid those micro scratches that can lead to wrinkles and blemishes. A high quality set will cost more, but it is well worth the investment.

239.   Rub your feet down with the Vaseline before bed and leave it on. Cover your feet with socks to protect your bedding when you go to sleep. The next morning you will awaken to softer feet.

240.   Watch video tutorials to get makeup tips. You no longer have to be a makeup artist to make your face look beautiful. All you simply need to do is to find any video sharing site and

you'll find step-by-step tutorials on how to create any number of looks with makeup.

241.   If you desire to emphasize your gorgeous deep green or hazel eyes, use colors that will highlight these colors in a way that they look like candlelight. These could include deep wines, shimmery purples, frosty gunmetal gray, or lighter golden brown tones.

242.   Keep moisturizer handy to keep your skin looking vibrant. Particularly in winter, skin cracks and breaks and creates an undesirable appearance. When you moisturize, you are able to prevent the dry skin that leads to cracks.

243.   Make your shampoo and conditioner last longer. If you are using an expensive shampoo or conditioner that is thick, you can stretch out the amount of use you get out of it by watering it down. Be careful not to add too much water because this can ruin it.

244.   You can adjust your hair's cut and color to slim a fuller face. Styles that are longer and add length to the face will help. Opt for a hair length that lays somewhere between the chin and shoulders, but no shorter than the chin. Color around the face through high- or low-lights can

frame it. This is a good thing and you will focus on your positive features.

245.   Use a teabag piece to protect a fingernail that rips off. First, empty a teabag of its leaves. Then, cut out a piece of the teabag in the shape of your nail to provide coverage. Then put the trimmed out piece over the tear, and use a clear nail polish to paint over the whole thing.

246.   Avoid commercial "body butters" that contain chemicals, dyes and additives. All natural walnut oil or peanut oil make wonderful all-over body moisturizers. They are very inexpensive and are scent free. If you want scent, you can add the essential oil of your choice. After your bath, slather walnut or peanut oil on lavishly. Wrap up in an old terry-cloth robe and curl up with a good book or a movie while your moisture treatment soaks in.

247.   Apply a lotion or cream containing sunscreen every day. You have to live your whole life with the same skin and it is worth the investment to protect it. You should start off each day with a coat of sunscreen before you even think of going outside. Your skin will thank you.

248.   Consider using a purple eye shadow, rather than black or brown. Black and brown can be boring. Purple can really make your eyes pop. Purple eyeshadow is not as bold as you might think. From a distance, it will look like a black or a brown. Even so, it will give your eyes a little extra something.

249.   Make sure that your blush and your lip color are in harmony. If you are using blush, it is important to make sure that it matches the color you are using for your lips. Pink should be with pink, red with red, etc. If the colors vary too greatly from one another, they will clash terribly.

250.   Here is a beauty tip! Warm your concealer before using it! Often when you put concealer on it can come off looking thick and caked. You have to know how to conceal your concealer. First warm it by rubbing it in circular motion on the back of your hand! Then use your finger to apply.

251.   If you have dry skin, or older looking skin, you need to be exfoliating on a weekly basis. You should also do this if you are applying any kind of tanning lotion. You want to exfoliate first to get the most out of the tanning lotion you are using.

252.   To get smaller pores, cut refined sugars from your diet. Eating large amounts of refined sugar enlarges your pores, and can also lead to breakouts. If you have a sweet tooth, try sating your cravings with natural sugars like the ones found in fruit. Your skin will definitely thank you for it!

253.   Exfoliating your body prior to applying tanning lotion or spending time in a tanning bed will extend the life of your tan! Since skin sheds, it's best to do as much of it as possible before getting that great tan so you can keep the glorious glow even longer! Any natural exfoliant applied a day or two before tanning will do!

254.   If you haven't taken care of your physical appearance for a long time, don't be scared off by the amount of work it takes to improve it. Although the initial time investment might be high it is much easier to maintain a good appearance than to initially create it.

255.   If you have grey hair dyed dark, and your roots are beginning to show, try putting the same color mascara as your dyed hair. If your hair is dyed a lighter color such as blond, spray some hairspray on the roots and use a bit of bronze or

gold-colored eyeshadow. Or, you can try one of the root color-combs available at local beauty supply stores.

256.   You may not have stuck your finger in an electrical socket, but your hair frizzes might suggest you had. To tame these nasty beasts, you will want to add moisture to your hair. Stay away from hairspray as it has alcohol that dries the hair. Apply hair serum to damp hair to lock in the moisture, and keep uncontrolled hair at bay.

257.   Believe it or not, you can reduce the puffy look of your face from within. Place an ice cube in your mouth, and press it against the roof with your tongue. Follow it up with splashes of cold water on the outside and within minutes, without spending a fortune, you have a quick and effective remedy!

258.   Before bed, put a little natural oil, such as walnut oil, on your eyebrows. This can improve the look of your eyebrows by making the hair look glossier. Vaseline can cause unsightly acne, so try not to get it elsewhere on your face.

259.   Cracked heels and dry, flaking feet are very unattractive, especially in sandals. To combat this problem, right before you go to bed, soak your

feet in a warm water bath for ten minutes, coat them with petroleum jelly and then cover them with a thick pair of socks to lock in the moisture. In no time, you'll have soft feet.

260.   If the idea of applying strips of false lashes gives you cold feet, consider single lashes instead. These are considerably easier to apply and require only a small amount of eyelash glue, compared with the amount used for full lashes. Individual lashes, when placed in the outer corner of the eyes, produce a far more natural effect.

261.   Always apply a heat protectant spray to your hair before using a curling iron, flat iron or hair dryer. Heat can damage your hair, leaving it brittle, dry and full of split ends. Just like their name implies, heat protectant sprays coat your hair to protect it from the heat. This allows it to stay smooth, sleek and shiny no matter how you choose to style your hair.

262.   Remove the arch from your eyebrows if you have a problem with dark circles under your eyes. The arch in your eyebrows can create a circular look around your eyes. This can exaggerate any dark circles you might already

have. To remedy this, just tweeze your eyebrows so that they are straighter.

263.   Start wearing shimmer eye shadow. This type of eye shadow gives your eyes a shine that brightens your eyes and gives them the illusion of being bigger. When you are choosing the shade of shimmer eye shadow, it's best to choose a shade that is within a shade of two of your own skin. Have fun trying out various application techniques and colors.

264.   If your favorite color nail polish is getting empty and a bit tacky, add a few drops of nail polish remover to give it new life! You don't have to throw away a half empty bottle of nail lacquer, just mix in a small amount of regular remover, shake well and your old polish will work like new again.

265.   Glossy lips look fuller. Use a liner and a brush to apply bronzer that is a few shades darker than your skin. Try putting on a top coat of gold, coral, or peach lip gloss.

266.   If you're in between hair dresser appointments, and need to hide some roots, use dark mascara on black or brunette hair and gold eye shadow on blond hair! Nobody is perfect and

if you've scheduled your hair salon appointment too far in advance to save your roots from showing, brush them lightly with appropriately colored mascara or combine hair spray and blond shades of powder to conceal those roots until you can see your stylist!

267.   To give more definition to your eyes apply mascara. If you only have a few minutes, you can apply mascara to highlight your eyes, and look like you have spent more time than you really have getting ready. Adding eye color will only take a few moments, and really completes your look.

268.   When you are trying to improve the quality of your skin, one point that you can never overlook in your routine is a good exfoliation. You should do this at least twice a week and you should have a separate product for your face and your body. These will help to make your skin look younger.

269.   For soft feet, apply lotion or Vaseline and wrap in cling wrap before going to bed. You should then put socks on your feet. You should do this at least once a week for the softest feet. This will prepare even the driest feet for summer and wearing sandals.

270.   Tint your eyebrows. This can be done with a simple eye and brow pencil every time that you apply your makeup, or you can go to a salon and have them tinted with a permanent dye. Nice eyebrows provide facial definition and help you appear awake and aware.

271.   Before using any kind of eyelash glue around your eyes, test it on the inside of your arm twenty-four hours before you are planning to apply it to your eyes. This is the best way to test for allergies and can help you avoid having your eyes swell shut from an allergic reaction.

272.   There are some things that should be avoided after waxing. Do not go into direct sunlight or visit a tanning bed for at least twenty-four hours. Also, stay out of the shower if possible. This can be problematic due to the fact that your pores are completely open. You will achieve a better result if you wait.

273.   If one likes wearing accessories when they are getting ready to go out for the day then getting a piercing can be appealing. However if one is concerned about enhancing their beauty then they should think carefully about where they want their piercing. Having too many

piercings or piercings in weird places can scare people away.

274.   If you are trying to reduce the puffiness around your eyes try holding a cold spoon on the puffy areas. The cold can cause the puffiness to go away making your face look more beautiful.

275.   If you have fine lines around your eyes, mouth, and forehead, you should look for cosmetics with light-reflecting particles. These products, which are just more matte than shimmery, can reflect light in a way that appears to make the fine lines simply disappear. You can use this trick all over your face, or just in your laugh lines.

276.   If you have a square-shaped face, create a softer look by applying a cream-based rose, pink or coral blush. Use your fingers to apply the cream to your cheeks. Next, use a gentle, pulling motion to blend the color up towards your temples.

277.   If you are looking for some individualized attention from a cosmetics salesperson, visit the mall or department store during the early morning or daytime during the week. If you go on the weekend, your consultant will not be able

to give you a thorough assessment and unhurried cosmetics application.

278.   Try to avoid very hot water when showering or bathing. Hot water makes your pores open too much, letting important oils get out. You then are likely to wash them away. You can help keep your skin soft and beautiful by using warm or tepid water while washing. Cooler baths and showers will also save money on your energy bills.

279.   To make your eyelashes look thicker, dust them with a coat of loose powder before applying your mascara. Use a small brush to apply a thin layer of translucent powder to your eyelashes, taking care not to get the powder in your eyes. Follow up with a coat of your favorite mascara over the top of the powder.

280.   Remove the arch from your eyebrows if you have a problem with dark circles under your eyes. The arch in your eyebrows can create a circular look around your eyes. This can exaggerate any dark circles you might already have. To remedy this, just tweeze your eyebrows so that they are straighter.

281.   A great tip to use when tweezing your eyebrows is to use restrain. Over plucking the brows can lead to bald patches and emaciated brows where hair only grows back irregularly. If this has happened, use a brow gel which is protein-spiked to encourage healthy regrowth and brow fillers that can shade in areas that are problems.

282.   Create a funky, modern nail design by using scrapbooking scissors with scalloped, zig-zag or other edges. You can cut regular cellophane tape with the scissors and place them on your nails before painting to create great stripes, two-tone effects, or other interesting designs. Try using matte polishes next to glossy ones for a multi-textured effect.

283.   Pineapple can be a great food to help you lose weight and look great! This fruit contains bromelain in addition to being sweet and delicious. This is a digestive enzyme that helps with the processing of fats, proteins and starches. Improving digestion can speed up your metabolism.

284.   Once you have found a haircolor you like, be sure to buy an extra box or two of it to keep at home. That way, you will never be out of the

color you like if they happen to run out of it at the local drugstore or beauty center.

285.   When going to the beach, use this trick to make your waist look narrower. With a white pencil liner, dot the shape of an egg on both sides, starting just below the rib cage. Then fill the egg area with a little self-tanner just one shade darker than your natural skin tone and blend it in.

286.   Add some gloss or color to your lips. Applying tinted lip gloss to your lips helps to give your lips a soft, finished look. If you are looking to draw more attention to your lips, add lipstick or lip stain. By adding either one of these it will help to improve your overall look.

287.   Remove dead skin cells and shave prior to using any spray tan product. Proper skin preparation ensures an even coating of color, making the end result look more natural.

288.   To keep from getting eye bags, drink plenty of water before you go to bed. One of the leading causes of eyebags is dehydration during the night. If you still have eyebags when you wake up, rest cold, caffeinated teabags on your

eyes for about 10 minutes. This will nourish your eyes and make the bags disappear.

289.   Many people tend to get dead skin on their lips. This makes them look old and dry. A great way to prevent this from happening is to brush your lips gently with a toothbrush every single day. After you have done this, you will want to put some balm on to keep them protected.

290.   Keep some fabric softener sheets on hand for beauty emergencies. Fabric sheets can be used to tame a static skirt that wants to stick you your hose. It can do the same for wild hair. Another thing it is good for is running through your hair to quell obnoxious odors like smoke.

291.   Use steam to refresh your face. Steam releases the impurities in your pores, and you don't need to go to a sauna. A bowl or other container of hot water and a towel are all you need; just hold your head over it and let the piping hot steam redeem your skin.

292.   Always wash your face using a mild cleanser once or twice per day, no matter what your skin type is. Just remember to rinse off all of your makeup prior to using such a cleanser. If you do

not do this you may clog your pores and get pimples.

293. As you get older, exfoliation becomes more and more important to your skin. Use a glycolic acid-rich cream, facial scrub, or even a retinoid gel to slough off the top layer pf dead skin cells and to reveal the fresh, radiant new skin cells beneath. This can be done three to four times per week for the best effect.

294. Cracked heels and dry, flaking feet are very unattractive, especially in sandals. To combat this problem, right before you go to bed, soak your feet in a warm water bath for ten minutes, coat them with petroleum jelly and then cover them with a thick pair of socks to lock in the moisture. In no time, you'll have soft feet.

295. To make small eyes appear larger, try lining your lower waterline with a white or peach colored eyeliner. By lightening the color of your waterline so it blends better with the white part of your eye, you can create the illusion that your eyes are larger and brighter than they really are.

296. If you use a blow dryer to style your hair, use a styling product that protects your hair from the heat. You can find this type of product in the

beauty section of Target or Walmart or even at Sally Beauty Supply. This spray is great at helping hair dry faster while preventing split ends. The formula in the protectant will keep your hair hydrated and smelling wonderful!

297.   Consuming large quantities of water each day can help you keep your skin looking great without having to buy expensive products. Water naturally helps cleanse your body of toxins, and this action provides you with beautiful and clear skin throughout the day.

298.   Only apply shimmer where light may enhance it. That means you get a nice glow effect. Use a highlighter on your nose, brows, and cheekbones. Cover this with a light layer of powder.

299.   Put on lip balm every day. Lip balm is an essential ingredient in keeping your lips beautiful. You should apply it to your lips at night when you go to bed, and in the morning before you put any lipstick or gloss on your lips. Your lips will stay looking younger and fuller.

300.   Fruit juice just might be your secret weapon in the fight for better-looking skin. A daily intake of essential nutrients found in fruits and

vegetables will benefit your entire body, including your skin. Juices made from fresh fruit are a healthy, fresh way to incorporate fruit into your diet. Simply replacing sweet drinks, such as soda, will drastically improve your skin's texture and moisture.

301.   Separate products for softening, protecting, and coloring are no longer necessary! Try using a tinted moisturizer instead of a typical foundation. You can save yourself a lot of time and money buying a lightly tinted moisturizer with a sunscreen to replace the heavier old-fashioned foundations and creams.

302.   Paint your toenails before you go to bed. Make sure you have given your nail polish plenty of time to dry before going to bed. When you shower in the morning you can easily peel off any excess polish that you get on your toes for that perfect manicured look.

303.   Once you are finished putting on your lipstick, put your finger in your mouth and then pull the skin out to form an "O" shape. By doing this you will ensure you do not get lipstick on your pearly whites.

304.   When attempting to improve your appearance, the most important things to keep in mind are your clothes, posture, skin, and fitness. Enhancing these features can help to improve your overall look.

305.   An excellent suggestion for achieving full lips is trying a glossy look. Dip a concealer brush into a bronzer that is a couple of shades darker than your skin tone, and outline your lips with it. Pick a gold, peach or coral gloss to finish the look.

306.   Avoid using hot tools on hair every couple days to encourage the growth of strong and healthy hair. Curling irons, straighteners, and blow dryers can cause breakage and significant damage to your hair. Not using these tools for a few days every week will give your hair time to recover.

307.   To get rid of white patches on your nails, consume more calcium. The patches are a sign of vitamin deficiency. Clearing up those white spots will allow you to get a smoother and more consistent look with your nail polish. If you can't add more calcium to your diet, start taking a supplement.

308.   If you find that your feet are dry and scaly looking and feeling, try using a petroleum jelly product to treat them. Apply a generous amount on your feet and cover them with thick socks at night before you go to bed. Your feet will absorb the moisture out of the petroleum jelly and will quickly look and feel much better.

309.   Think about using eyelash extensions. This is an excellent suggestion for women who are attending formal events. The end result is a brighter, younger look. You'll be very pleased with your appearance.

310.   A great way to make small eyes appear to look much bigger is to steer clear of dark shades of eye shadow. Begin by using a nude base as a foundation, and then use a shadow that is one or two shades darker than the foundation in the crease. After blend the color up towards the brow by using your finger.

311.   Fill a tiny sample jar or empty pot of lip gloss with your favorite moisturizer. You can place this portable container in your car, at your desk drawer, purse or even in your travel bag. Use a small amount of moisturizer any time you feel like your skin is getting dry.

312.   Check to see if you are allergic to fake eyelashes before using them. Test for a reaction by placing a small amount of glue on the back of your arm. Protect the test area with a piece of gauze or cloth.

313.   If you don't like the look of your hair curled with a curling iron, try curling it with a straightener. Simply wrap your hair around the straightener and pull it through to the ends. This produces a much more natural looking curl, although it can take a little longer to do.

314.   Before putting on your favorite sandals for the summer season, take the time to moisturize your feet using Vaseline. Before bed, slather your feet with a thick layer of Vaseline and cover them with an old pair of socks. As you sleep, the Vaseline will penetrate thick, calloused skin, helping to eliminate cracks and dryness. The next morning when you remove the socks, your feet will be soft and supple so you can wear your favorite sandals with pride.

315.   If you continually get acne only on one side of your face, it could be caused by your cell phone. Make sure you clean your cell phone regularly to remove dirt and oil. You may also want to try switching sides each time you talk on

the phone to give the acne-prone side of your face a break.

316.   It does not matter how tired or pressed for time you may be, you should never skip your cleansing rituals. Drier skin benefits from thick, creamy cleansers, whereas oily skin benefits most from cleansing balms, washes, or bars. All skin types can be dulled by buildup of makeup, sweat, and dead skin cells.

317.   Keep a few particular beauty products in your fridge. In summertime, this can be extra helpful. Keeping your make up in your fridge will allow you to use it regardless of the weather. Keeping them cool will also give you skin some relief in hot temperatures.

318.   If the idea of applying strips of false lashes gives you cold feet, consider single lashes instead. These are considerably easier to apply and require only a small amount of eyelash glue, compared with the amount used for full lashes. Individual lashes, when placed in the outer corner of the eyes, produce a far more natural effect.

319.   Even the most skilled makeup artist sometimes has difficulty applying lipstick neatly.

After you have applied it, use a cleanup brush that has been dipped in powder to place the powder all along the lip outline. Next, use a disposable wedge sponge to blot away any excess powder that may be left.

320.   Keep to a schedule for maximum beauty benefit. You do not have to schedule everything, but you do need to schedule your meals. Studies have shown that people who are consistent with their routines concerning food and drink, look years younger, and live longer, than people who are sporadic with their eating times.

321.   Separate products for softening, protecting, and coloring are no longer necessary! Try using a tinted moisturizer instead of a typical foundation. You can save yourself a lot of time and money buying a lightly tinted moisturizer with a sunscreen to replace the heavier old-fashioned foundations and creams.

322.   To help your lip gloss last longer, apply lip liner first. Fill in your whole lip with the liner before putting on your gloss. With the liner applied, the gloss will have something to stick to, which will help it stay on all day long. For the best effect, use a liner close to the natural color of your lip.

323.   Slice a potato into thin strips. By putting this on your eyes, you can reduce puffiness. Keep the potato slice on your eye fr roughly ten minutes. If not potatoes, you can use cucumber, cool teaspoons, or teabags. This eliminates the puffy look and helps you looked more alert and revived in no time.

324.   Sometimes, when coloring your hair, you may find that the color you chose simply isn't strong or intense enough for your liking. You can solve this problem by purchasing a second box of color, mixing half the product with shampoo, and reapplying it to just-colored hair. Let it sit for only 5-10 minutes before rinsing and you will find the color intensified.

325.   UVA rays are as powerful in the wintertime as they are during the summer, so they need to be using a sunblock with an SPF of at least 15, no matter what season it is. This will allow your skin to remain protected against cancer and wrinkles too.

326.   Always exfoliate and shave before you use any spray on tanning products. Proper preparation of the skin before the application

will allow the color to spread more evenly, and that gives your skin a more natural appearance.

327.   Love the feel of waxing but hate the pain? When waxing at home, a half hour before doing the wax, apply a tooth-numbing cream to the areas that are going to be waxed. This will numb the skin temporarily and make the waxing much less painful yet will not damage or hurt your skin.

328.   Apply a moisturizer that is light before putting a fake tan on your skin. A fake tan will collect on spots of your skin that are dry. You should make sure you pay attention to your feet, elbows, knees and around your wrists. Apply lotion to these areas before applying a fake tanner.

329.   Make your hair smell good. Spritz your favorite perfume on your hairbrush or comb and brush your hair. This will give your hair a great and lasting scent. If you notice the scent is fading, do it again. Knowing your hair smells good can make you feel better about it.

330.   Never go to the cosmetics counter for skincare application tips while your skin is irritated, bumpy, or in especially bad shape. Applying a new cosmetic product over the

irritated skin can actually make the condition much worse. Wait until the condition has improved, then make the trip and set up an appointment.

331.   Always apply a heat protectant spray to your hair before using a curling iron, flat iron or hair dryer. Heat can damage your hair, leaving it brittle, dry and full of split ends. Just like their name implies, heat protectant sprays coat your hair to protect it from the heat. This allows it to stay smooth, sleek and shiny no matter how you choose to style your hair.

332.   Peppermint oil mixed with water makes a really good, natural and alcohol free mouthwash. Add a single drop of peppermint oil for each ounce of water used. You want to make sure the water is boiled first and then measure the oil into a ceramic container. Add boiling water for the next step. Cover the container with a clean cloth (i.e. a handkerchief) and allow to cool. Pour the mixture into a sterile bottle and tightly screw on the lid. Now you have mouthwash!

333.   Give your face a monthly beauty treatment. You do not need to go to a spa to get your skin in its best shape. You can, instead, give yourself a complete facial at home. Start with a product to

exfoliate, follow with a mudpack, next apply an astringent, and finish with a deep moisturizer.

334.   Keep to a schedule for maximum beauty benefit. You do not have to schedule everything, but you do need to schedule your meals. Studies have shown that people who are consistent with their routines concerning food and drink, look years younger, and live longer, than people who are sporadic with their eating times.

335.   People who have fair skin and hair need a little extra tinting to bring out definition. The best is to use eyebrow tinting, this will bring out the color of your eyebrows as well as add an extra pop to your eyes. Sometimes the subtle little things can make the most difference.

336.   A great tip to use when tweezing your eyebrows is to use restrain. Over plucking the brows can lead to bald patches and emaciated brows where hair only grows back irregularly. If this has happened, use a brow gel which is protein-spiked to encourage healthy regrowth and brow fillers that can shade in areas that are problems.

337.   To get a smoother look when applying your eyeshadow, apply primer first. Primer will give

the eyeshadow an even surface and will create a smooth effect. It will also make your eyeshadow color look brighter and more vibrant. Be sure to choose a primer specifically designed for use on the eyes.

338.　If you're in between hair dresser appointments, and need to hide some roots, use dark mascara on black or brunette hair and gold eye shadow on blond hair! Nobody is perfect and if you've scheduled your hair salon appointment too far in advance to save your roots from showing, brush them lightly with appropriately colored mascara or combine hair spray and blond shades of powder to conceal those roots until you can see your stylist!

339.　Using Vaseline on your eyebrows and eyelashes is going to have a couple different benefits. If you use it at night before you go to bed, you are going to benefit by having lashes and brows that are much shinier. If you use the Vaseline to prep for brow liner, you will notice that your brows will stay in place better.

340.　Never ever go to bed with your makeup on your face. This causes more damage than just ruining a good pillow case. Your pores will get extremely clogged and you will suffer many blemishes. Taking the time to wash your face each night will surely benefit you for many years.

341.   Use a high quality, waterproof mascara at the beach or swimming pool. Water can quickly wash away your beauty routine. Using waterproof products can keep this from happening. If all of your other products wash off but your mascara remains, you will still look "done up" and complete.

342.   Guacamole with avocado is a delicious treat, but are you aware of its amazing softening properties to your skin? Get yourself a ripe avocado that has the skin and pit taken out. Mash it up in a bowl. Let the mixture set on your entire body for 20 minutes and rinse away. Avocado is a natural moisturizer, so it will make your skin very soft.

343.   Learning what is appropriate and what is not appropriate as far as what to wear can be a big part of beauty. While flaunting one's assets is not a bad thing, there is the problem of not knowing how much is too much. Dressing in a manner that is too revealing can make others think poorly of you and disregard any beauty.